Beginners Guide to Romantic Sex

15+ Tips for Couples to Make Sex More Romantic and Intimate

Cheryl Bach

Beginners Guide to Romantic Sex

Cheryl Bach

Table of Contents

I.

Introduction

A. Why Romance and Intimacy Matter in Sex

Think about what makes sex special between two people who love each other. It's not just about physical pleasure. It's the emotional connection—the feelings of love, closeness, and trust—that make it meaningful. This emotional side of sex is what we call romance and intimacy.

Romance is like the spark that ignites a fire. It's the little gestures—like holding hands, giving compliments, or cuddling—that show love and affection. Intimacy, on the other hand, is about feeling close and connected to your partner. It's sharing your thoughts, fears, and dreams with each other.

Why are romance and intimacy so important? Well, they're the glue that holds a relationship together. Couples who feel loved and connected are happier and more satisfied with their relationship. And when you feel close to your partner, sex becomes more than just a physical act—it becomes a way to express your love and deepen your bond.

B. What This Book Is All About

This book is for couples who want to make their sex life more romantic and intimate. Whether you're just starting out in a relationship or you've been together for years, there's always room to make things even better between the sheets.

In this book, we'll give you practical tips and ideas for adding more romance and intimacy to your sex life. From setting the mood to trying new things together, we'll cover everything you need to know to make sex more than just a routine. So if you're ready to spice things up and bring the spark back into your relationship, this book is for you.

II.

Understanding the Importance of Romance in Sex

A. Link between Romance and Intimacy

When we think about romance and intimacy, they often go hand in hand, especially in the context of sexual relationships. Romance is like the gentle breeze that carries the fragrance of love, while intimacy is the warm embrace that makes us feel cherished and understood. Together, they create a powerful synergy that enriches our connection with our partners and deepens our experience of sex.

At the core of the link between romance and intimacy lies the notion of emotional connection. Romance is about expressing love and desire through thoughtful gestures, such as sweet words, tender touches, or surprise gifts. These acts of romance not only show our partners that we care but also strengthen the emotional bond between us. And when we feel emotionally connected to our partners, it naturally enhances the intimacy we experience during sex.

Intimacy, on the other hand, is about feeling close and vulnerable with our partners. It's the sense of trust and openness that allows us to share our deepest thoughts, fears, and desires without fear of judgment. When we feel intimate with our partners, we're more likely to let our guard down and fully immerse ourselves in the moment during sex, leading to a more fulfilling and satisfying experience.

In essence, romance and intimacy are two sides of the same coin—they both contribute to the emotional connection that makes sex meaningful and fulfilling. By nurturing romance and intimacy in our relationships, we create a strong foundation for intimacy that can withstand the test of time.

B. The Impact of Romance on Overall Relationship Satisfaction

Romance isn't just about making grand gestures or sweeping someone off their feet; it's about consistently showing love and appreciation for our partners in everyday moments. And when we prioritize romance in our relationships, it has a profound impact on our overall relationship satisfaction.

Studies have consistently shown that couples who engage in romantic behaviors, such as expressing gratitude, showing affection, and going on dates, report higher levels of relationship satisfaction and commitment. This is because romance helps to keep the spark alive and reminds us of the love and connection we share with our partners.

Moreover, romance isn't just beneficial for the individuals in the relationship—it also strengthens the relationship as a whole. When partners feel loved and appreciated, they're more likely to be supportive, understanding, and empathetic towards each other, leading to a more harmonious and fulfilling relationship overall.

But romance isn't just about the grand gestures—it's also about the little things we do for each other every day. Whether it's leaving a love note, cooking a special meal, or simply saying "I love you," these small acts of romance add up over time and contribute to the overall satisfaction and happiness we experience in our relationships.

C. Debunking Common Myths about Romantic Sex

Despite the undeniable importance of romance in sex, there are many myths and misconceptions surrounding the topic that can hinder our ability to cultivate romance in our relationships. Let's take a moment to debunk some of these myths:

Myth #1: Romance is only for special occasions.

Reality: Romance is not limited to anniversaries or Valentine's Day. It's about finding joy and connection in everyday moments and making our partners feel loved and appreciated on a regular basis.

Myth #2: Romance requires grand gestures.

Reality: While grand gestures can be nice, romance is more about the thought and effort behind the gesture rather than its scale. Simple acts of kindness and affection can be just as meaningful as extravagant displays of affection.

Myth #3: Romance fades over time.

Reality: While it's true that the initial passion of a new relationship may fade over time, romance can actually deepen and evolve as the relationship matures. It's about finding new ways to show love and appreciation for our partners as we grow together.

By understanding the importance of romance in sex and debunking common myths surrounding the topic, we can cultivate more fulfilling and intimate relationships with our partners. So let's embrace romance in all its forms and create lasting memories of love and connection in our relationships.

III.

Building Emotional Connection

A. Communication: Key to Fostering Emotional Intimacy

Communication is the cornerstone of any healthy relationship, and when it comes to building emotional intimacy, it plays a crucial role. Effective communication allows couples to express their thoughts, feelings, and desires openly and honestly, creating a safe space for vulnerability and connection.

One of the key aspects of communication in fostering emotional intimacy is active listening. This means truly paying attention to what your partner is saying, without interrupting or judging. It involves not only hearing their words but also understanding their emotions and perspective. By practicing active listening, couples can deepen their understanding of each other and strengthen their emotional bond.

Another important aspect of communication is expressing appreciation and gratitude. Taking the time to acknowledge and validate our partner's feelings and efforts can go a long way in building trust and connection. Whether it's a simple "thank you" for doing the dishes or a heartfelt expression of love, these words of affirmation can nurture feelings of closeness and intimacy.

Finally, communication also involves being able to express our own needs and boundaries. This requires vulnerability and honesty, as it means opening up about our desires, fears, and insecurities. By sharing our innermost thoughts and feelings with our partner, we invite them into our emotional world and create opportunities for deeper connection and understanding.

B. Prioritizing Quality Time Together

In today's fast-paced world, it's easy for couples to get caught up in the hustle and bustle of daily life and neglect their relationship. However, prioritizing quality time together is essential for building emotional intimacy and maintaining a strong connection.

Quality time doesn't necessarily mean extravagant dates or expensive vacations; it's about carving out moments of undivided attention and genuine connection with your partner. Whether it's sharing a meal together, going for a walk in the park, or simply cuddling on the couch, these small moments of togetherness can strengthen the bond between couples and deepen their emotional connection.

It's also important to make time for meaningful conversations and shared activities. This means putting away distractions like phones and TVs and focusing on each other fully. By engaging in open and honest dialogue and participating in activities that bring joy and fulfillment, couples can create lasting memories and foster a sense of closeness and intimacy.

C. Cultivating Trust and Vulnerability

Trust and vulnerability are essential ingredients in building emotional intimacy, as they create a foundation of safety and security in a relationship. When partners feel safe to be themselves and express their true thoughts and feelings without fear of judgment or rejection, it fosters a deep sense of connection and closeness.

One way to cultivate trust and vulnerability is by being reliable and consistent in our actions. This means following through on our promises, being there for our partner in times of need, and being honest and transparent in our communication. By demonstrating reliability and integrity, we show our partner that they can depend on us, which strengthens their trust and confidence in the relationship.

Vulnerability, on the other hand, involves being open and authentic about our innermost thoughts, feelings, and experiences. It means allowing ourselves to be seen and heard, even when it feels scary or uncomfortable. By sharing our vulnerabilities with our partner, we invite them into our emotional world and create opportunities for deeper connection and understanding.

Ultimately, building emotional connection requires a willingness to be present, open, and vulnerable with our partner. By prioritizing communication, quality time together, and cultivating trust and vulnerability, couples can create a strong foundation of emotional intimacy that enhances their sexual relationship and strengthens their bond.

Cheryl Bach

IV.

Creating a Romantic Atmosphere

A. Setting the Mood

The ambiance plays a significant role in setting the stage for a romantic and intimate sexual experience. Creating the right atmosphere can heighten arousal, increase relaxation, and deepen emotional connection between partners. Whether you're in the comfort of your own home, a cozy hotel room, or out in nature, the ambiance sets the tone for a memorable and satisfying encounter.

First and foremost, consider the lighting. Soft, dim lighting is often ideal for creating a romantic atmosphere. Candles, fairy lights, or strategically placed lamps can help to create a warm and inviting glow that enhances intimacy without being too harsh or bright. Avoid harsh overhead lights or fluorescent lighting, as they can be distracting and disrupt the mood.

Next, consider the decor and surroundings. Choose fabrics, colors, and textures that evoke feelings of comfort and sensuality. Soft, luxurious bedding, plush pillows, and silky fabrics can add a touch of luxury and indulgence to the space. Personal touches such as photos, artwork, or mementos that hold sentimental value can also help to create a sense of intimacy and connection.

Finally, pay attention to the overall ambiance and energy of the space. Consider factors such as temperature, cleanliness, and clutter, as these can all impact the mood and comfort level of both partners. Creating a clean, clutter-free environment that is warm and inviting will help to ensure that both partners feel relaxed and comfortable, allowing them to fully immerse themselves in the experience.

B. Incorporating Sensory Experiences

Creating a romantic atmosphere isn't just about what you see—it's about engaging all five senses to heighten arousal and enhance intimacy. By incorporating sensory experiences into your environment, you can create a multi-dimensional experience that stimulates both the body and mind.

Start by considering the sense of sight. Choose visually pleasing elements such as soft lighting, beautiful decor, and romantic artwork to create an aesthetically pleasing environment. Consider incorporating candles, fairy lights, or a flickering fireplace to add warmth and intimacy to the space.

Next, think about the sense of sound. Soft music, nature sounds, or even the sound of your partner's voice can help to create a soothing and sensual atmosphere. Choose music that is calming and relaxing, or opt for a playlist of your favorite romantic songs to set the mood.

The sense of touch is also crucial in creating a romantic atmosphere. Soft, comfortable bedding, plush pillows, and luxurious fabrics can enhance tactile sensations and make partners feel pampered and indulged. Consider incorporating sensual touches such as silk scarves, feather ticklers, or massage oils to add an extra layer of intimacy to the experience.

Don't forget about the sense of smell. Scented candles, essential oils, or fragrant flowers can help to create a romantic ambiance and stimulate the olfactory senses. Choose scents that are soothing and sensual, such as lavender, vanilla, or jasmine, to create a calming and inviting environment.

Finally, consider the sense of taste. Indulge in sensual treats such as chocolate-covered strawberries, champagne, or exotic fruits to tantalize the taste buds and add an element of luxury to the experience. Experiment with different flavors and textures to create a sensory feast that delights all the senses.

C. Practical Tips for Creating a Romantic Environment in Various Settings

Creating a romantic environment doesn't have to be limited to the confines of your home. Whether you're planning a romantic getaway in a hotel room, a picnic in the park, or a cozy night under the stars, there are plenty of ways to create a romantic atmosphere in any setting.

At home, you have the freedom to customize your environment to suit your preferences. Consider transforming your bedroom into a romantic retreat with soft lighting, luxurious bedding, and sensual decor. Create a cozy nook with blankets and pillows where you can cuddle up together and enjoy each other's company.

If you're planning a romantic getaway in a hotel room, take advantage of the amenities available to you. Request a room with a view, a Jacuzzi tub, or a balcony where you can enjoy the scenery together. Bring along some candles, music, and sensual treats to create a romantic atmosphere in your temporary home away from home.

For outdoor adventures, consider packing a picnic basket with your favorite snacks, drinks, and a cozy blanket. Find a secluded spot where you can enjoy the beauty of nature together, whether it's a scenic overlook, a secluded beach, or a quiet forest clearing. Take in the sights, sounds, and smells of the natural world as you connect with your partner in a romantic and intimate setting.

No matter where you are, the key to creating a romantic environment is to focus on the details that matter most to you and your partner. Whether it's soft lighting, soothing music, or sensual touches, take the time to set the stage for a memorable and intimate experience that brings you closer together.

Cheryl Bach

V.

Enhancing Physical Intimacy

A. Different Types of Physical Affection beyond Intercourse

Physical intimacy is about more than just sex—it encompasses a wide range of touch and affectionate gestures that can deepen the connection between partners. Exploring different types of physical affection beyond intercourse allows couples to express their love and desire in diverse ways, enriching their sexual relationship and fostering a deeper sense of intimacy.

One type of physical affection is kissing, which can range from gentle pecks on the lips to passionate make-out sessions. Kissing stimulates the release of oxytocin, a hormone that promotes bonding and connection, making it an essential component of physical intimacy.

Another form of physical affection is hugging, which involves wrapping your arms around your partner in a tight embrace. Hugging releases feel-good hormones like serotonin and dopamine, helping to reduce stress and increase feelings of happiness and connection.

Other forms of physical affection include holding hands, cuddling, and caressing each other's bodies. These acts of touch convey love, warmth, and comfort, strengthening the emotional bond between partners and enhancing their sense of intimacy.

By exploring different types of physical affection beyond intercourse, couples can discover new ways to connect with each other and deepen their physical and emotional intimacy.

B. Importance of Non-Sexual Touch and Cuddling

Non-sexual touch and cuddling play a crucial role in fostering emotional intimacy and strengthening the bond between partners. While sexual touch is focused on arousal and pleasure, non-sexual touch is about expressing love, comfort, and affection without the expectation of intercourse.

Cuddling, in particular, is a powerful form of non-sexual touch that promotes feelings of closeness and connection between partners. Whether it's spooning in bed, snuggling on the couch, or simply holding each other in a warm embrace, cuddling releases oxytocin and promotes feelings of trust, safety, and intimacy.

Non-sexual touch can also help to reduce stress, alleviate anxiety, and promote relaxation, making it an essential component of physical and emotional well-being. By engaging in regular cuddling sessions and non-sexual touch, couples can strengthen their bond and create a deeper sense of intimacy in their relationship.

C. Incorporating Massage and Sensual Touch into Your Routine

Massage and sensual touch are powerful tools for enhancing physical intimacy and arousal between partners. Whether it's a full-body massage, a foot rub, or a sensual caress, these forms of touch can stimulate the senses, increase relaxation, and heighten arousal, leading to more fulfilling and satisfying sexual experiences.

Massage, in particular, has numerous benefits for both physical and emotional well-being. It helps to relax tense muscles, improve circulation, and reduce stress and anxiety, creating a state of deep relaxation and arousal that is conducive to intimacy.

Sensual touch, on the other hand, focuses on stimulating erogenous zones and eliciting pleasurable sensations throughout the body. By exploring each other's bodies with curiosity and openness, partners can discover new erogenous zones and learn how to pleasure each other in ways that enhance arousal and intimacy.

Incorporating massage and sensual touch into your routine doesn't have to be complicated or intimidating. Start by setting aside time for regular massage sessions, either as a standalone activity or as part of foreplay before sex. Experiment with different techniques, pressures, and strokes to find what feels most pleasurable for you and your partner.

Remember, the key to incorporating massage and sensual touch into your routine is to approach it with an open mind and a spirit of exploration. By prioritizing physical intimacy and taking the time to pleasure each other with touch, couples can deepen their connection and create more fulfilling and satisfying sexual experiences together.

VI.
Spicing Up Foreplay

A. Understanding the Role of Foreplay in Enhancing Arousal and Intimacy

Foreplay is often referred to as the appetizer before the main course of sex, but its importance goes beyond mere preparation for intercourse. Foreplay plays a crucial role in enhancing arousal, building anticipation, and deepening emotional intimacy between partners.

Foreplay sets the stage for a more satisfying and pleasurable sexual experience by preparing both partners physically and mentally for sex. It helps to stimulate erogenous zones, increase blood flow to the genitals, and promote relaxation, making it easier to achieve and maintain arousal during intercourse.

But beyond its physical benefits, foreplay also serves as a powerful tool for building emotional intimacy and connection between partners. It provides an opportunity for couples to explore each other's bodies, communicate their desires and preferences, and deepen their bond through shared pleasure and intimacy.

By understanding the role of foreplay in enhancing arousal and intimacy, couples can learn to appreciate its importance and prioritize it as an essential part of their sexual routine.

B. Different Types of Foreplay Activities

Foreplay encompasses a wide range of activities that are designed to stimulate arousal, build anticipation, and enhance intimacy between partners. From tender kisses to sensual caresses to erotic massages, there are countless ways to explore and enjoy foreplay with your partner.

Kissing is often considered one of the most intimate forms of foreplay, as it allows partners to connect on a deep emotional and physical level. Whether it's gentle pecks on the lips, passionate make-out sessions, or exploring each other's mouths with tongues, kissing can be incredibly arousing and pleasurable for both partners.

Caressing and touching are also important aspects of foreplay, as they allow partners to explore each other's bodies and stimulate erogenous zones. Whether it's running your fingers through your partner's hair, tracing patterns on their skin, or gently massaging their muscles, tactile stimulation can be incredibly erotic and arousing.

Oral sex is another popular form of foreplay that can bring immense pleasure and excitement to both partners. Whether you're giving or receiving oral sex, the intimate act of pleasuring your partner with your mouth can be incredibly arousing and satisfying.

Other forms of foreplay include using sex toys, incorporating role play and fantasy, and exploring different positions and techniques. The key is to experiment with different activities and find what feels most pleasurable and exciting for you and your partner.

C. Communicating Desires and Preferences with Your Partner

Effective communication is essential for a fulfilling and satisfying sexual relationship, especially when it comes to foreplay. By openly discussing your desires, preferences, and boundaries with your partner, you can ensure that you both feel comfortable and confident in exploring new and exciting experiences together.

Start by having an honest and open conversation with your partner about what you enjoy and what you'd like to try during foreplay. This can involve discussing specific activities, techniques, or fantasies that you find arousing and pleasurable.

Be sure to listen to your partner's desires and preferences as well, and be willing to compromise and explore new things together. Remember that communication is a two-way street, and it's important to create a safe and non-judgmental space where both partners feel comfortable expressing their needs and desires.

In addition to verbal communication, pay attention to your partner's nonverbal cues and body language during foreplay. Notice how they respond to different touches, caresses, and kisses, and adjust your actions accordingly to ensure that they feel comfortable and pleasured.

By communicating openly and honestly with your partner, you can create a more fulfilling and satisfying sexual experience that deepens your emotional connection and strengthens your bond as a couple. So don't be afraid to speak up and share your desires—it's the key to unlocking a world of pleasure and intimacy in your relationship.

VII.
Trying New Things Together

A. Importance of Exploration and Experimentation in Keeping the Spark Alive

In any long-term relationship, it's natural for things to become routine and predictable over time. However, maintaining a healthy and satisfying sexual relationship requires a willingness to explore and experiment together. Trying new things can help to keep the spark alive, reignite passion, and deepen the connection between partners.

Exploration and experimentation allow couples to break out of their comfort zones, challenge assumptions, and discover new facets of their sexuality. Whether it's trying a new position, incorporating sex toys, or exploring role play and fantasy, the act of trying new things together can be incredibly exciting and rewarding.

Moreover, exploration and experimentation can help to increase arousal and excitement during sex by introducing novelty and unpredictability into the bedroom. By stepping outside of your usual routine and trying something new, you can create a sense of adventure and anticipation that enhances the overall experience for both partners.

B. Introducing Novelty into Your Sexual Routine

One of the keys to keeping the spark alive in a long-term relationship is to introduce novelty into your sexual routine. This can involve trying new activities, locations, or techniques that deviate from your usual patterns and routines.

Beginners Guide to Romantic Sex

One way to introduce novelty into your sexual routine is to explore different locations for sex. Whether it's in the bedroom, the living room, or even outdoors, changing up the environment can add excitement and spontaneity to your sexual encounters.

Another way to introduce novelty is to experiment with different positions and techniques. There are countless variations and combinations to try, so don't be afraid to get creative and explore what feels good for you and your partner.

You can also introduce novelty by incorporating sex toys and accessories into your play. From vibrators and dildos to bondage gear and massage oils, there are endless possibilities for adding excitement and variety to your sexual experiences.

C. Exploring Fantasies and Desires in a Safe and Respectful Manner

Fantasies and desires are a natural and healthy part of human sexuality, and exploring them with your partner can be an exciting and fulfilling experience. However, it's important to approach this exploration in a safe and respectful manner, ensuring that both partners feel comfortable and empowered throughout the process.

Start by having an open and honest conversation with your partner about your fantasies and desires. This can involve sharing specific fantasies, role-playing scenarios, or even discussing kinks and fetishes that you'd like to explore together.

It's important to approach this conversation with sensitivity and empathy, respecting your partner's boundaries and preferences at all times. Be prepared to listen nonjudgmentally and to communicate your own desires and boundaries as well.

Once you've identified shared fantasies and desires, you can begin to explore them together in a safe and consensual manner. This may involve setting boundaries, establishing safe words, and taking things slow to ensure that both partners feel comfortable and supported throughout the experience.

Remember, the goal of exploring fantasies and desires is to enhance intimacy and connection between partners, so always prioritize mutual respect, communication, and consent. By approaching this exploration with openness and respect, you can create a more fulfilling and satisfying sexual relationship that deepens your bond as a couple.

VIII.

Deepening Emotional Connection through Sex

A. Understanding the Emotional Aspects of Sexual Intimacy

Sexual intimacy is about more than just physical pleasure—it's also a powerful way to deepen emotional connection and strengthen the bond between partners. When approached with mindfulness and intention, sex can be a deeply intimate and transformative experience that nourishes the emotional connection between partners.

At its core, sexual intimacy involves vulnerability, trust, and mutual respect. It's about sharing not only our bodies but also our deepest thoughts, feelings, and desires with our partner. Through sex, we have the opportunity to express love, passion, and affection in ways that words alone cannot convey.

Sexual intimacy also has the potential to bring partners closer together emotionally by fostering feelings of closeness, connection, and belonging. The release of oxytocin, often referred to as the "love hormone," during sex promotes feelings of trust, bonding, and attachment, deepening the emotional connection between partners.

However, it's important to recognize that sexual intimacy can also bring up feelings of vulnerability, insecurity, and fear for some individuals. Past traumas, insecurities, and cultural or societal influences can impact our relationship with sex and intimacy, making it essential to approach sexual encounters with sensitivity, empathy, and understanding.

By understanding the emotional aspects of sexual intimacy, couples can cultivate a deeper appreciation for the transformative power of sex and harness its potential to strengthen their emotional connection.

B. Communicating Needs and Desires Openly and Honestly

Effective communication is essential for deepening emotional connection through sex. By openly and honestly communicating our needs, desires, and boundaries with our partner, we create a safe and supportive environment where both partners feel heard, valued, and respected.

Start by initiating a conversation with your partner about your sexual needs and desires. This can involve discussing specific preferences, fantasies, or areas of exploration that you'd like to explore together. Be sure to listen actively to your partner's needs and desires as well, and be open to finding common ground and compromise.

It's also important to communicate during sex itself, expressing what feels good, what doesn't, and any changes or adjustments you'd like to make. Use verbal and nonverbal cues to guide your partner and communicate your pleasure and satisfaction.

Additionally, don't be afraid to communicate about any concerns, fears, or insecurities you may have surrounding sex. Opening up about vulnerabilities can deepen emotional connection and foster a sense of trust and intimacy between partners.

Remember, effective communication is a two-way street, so be sure to create a safe and non-judgmental space where both partners feel comfortable expressing themselves openly and honestly.

C. Building Intimacy through Shared Sexual Experiences

Shared sexual experiences can be incredibly powerful tools for deepening emotional connection between partners. Whether it's exploring new fantasies and desires, trying new techniques and positions, or simply being present and attentive to each other's needs and desires, shared sexual experiences can create moments of deep intimacy and connection that strengthen the bond between partners.

One way to build intimacy through shared sexual experiences is to prioritize mutual pleasure and satisfaction. Focus on giving and receiving pleasure equally, and take the time to explore each other's bodies with curiosity, enthusiasm, and care.

Another way to build intimacy is to engage in activities that promote emotional connection and vulnerability during sex. This can involve maintaining eye contact, expressing love and affection verbally, or engaging in intimate acts of touch and caress that promote feelings of closeness and connection.

Finally, don't underestimate the power of aftercare in building intimacy after sex. Taking the time to cuddle, talk, and share your thoughts and feelings with each other can create a sense of emotional intimacy and connection that lingers long after the physical act of sex has ended.

By understanding the emotional aspects of sexual intimacy, communicating needs and desires openly and honestly, and building intimacy through shared sexual experiences, couples can deepen their emotional connection and strengthen their bond in profound and meaningful ways.

IX.

Overcoming Common Challenges

Sexual intimacy can face various challenges that can affect the romantic and intimate aspects of a relationship. In this chapter, we'll explore some common obstacles that couples may encounter and provide strategies for overcoming them.

A. Addressing Issues Such as Stress, Fatigue, and Lack of Time

Life can be hectic, and it's not uncommon for stress, fatigue, and lack of time to impact a couple's sex life. However, it's essential to prioritize intimacy and find ways to overcome these challenges to maintain a fulfilling sexual relationship.

Prioritize Self-Care: Take steps to manage stress and fatigue by prioritizing self-care practices such as exercise, meditation, and relaxation techniques. Taking care of your physical and mental well-being can help you feel more energized and present in your relationship.

Schedule Intimate Time: Set aside dedicated time for intimacy in your schedule, just like you would for any other important activity. This could involve scheduling regular date nights or intimate evenings at home where you can focus on connecting with your partner.

Get Creative: Find ways to make the most of the time you have together, even if it's limited. This could involve incorporating quick and easy intimacy boosters such as cuddling, kissing, or sensual massages into your daily routine.

B. Dealing with Communication Barriers and Insecurities

Communication is essential for a healthy and satisfying sexual relationship, but it's not always easy to talk about intimate topics. Communication barriers and insecurities can arise, making it challenging to address issues and express needs and desires effectively.

Create a Safe Space: Foster open and honest communication by creating a safe and non-judgmental space where both partners feel comfortable expressing themselves. Practice active listening and empathy to validate each other's feelings and experiences.

Practice Vulnerability: Be willing to be vulnerable and share your thoughts, feelings, and insecurities with your partner. Opening up about your fears and concerns can deepen emotional connection and foster intimacy in your relationship.

Seek Support: If communication barriers persist, consider seeking support from a couples therapist or counselor. A trained professional can provide guidance and tools to help you navigate difficult conversations and strengthen your communication skills.

C. Seeking Professional Help When Needed

Sometimes, challenges in a couple's sex life may require professional intervention to address underlying issues and find solutions. Seeking help from a qualified therapist or counselor can be instrumental in overcoming obstacles and restoring intimacy in the relationship.

Find a Qualified Professional: Look for a therapist or counselor who specializes in couples therapy or sex therapy and has experience working with issues related to intimacy and relationships.

Be Open to Therapy: Approach therapy with an open mind and a willingness to explore difficult topics and emotions. Remember that therapy is a collaborative process, and your therapist is there to support and guide you through the challenges you're facing.

Follow Through with Treatment: Commit to attending therapy sessions regularly and actively participating in the therapeutic process. Be open to trying new strategies and techniques recommended by your therapist and be patient with yourself and your partner as you work towards positive change.

By addressing common challenges such as stress, fatigue, and lack of time, dealing with communication barriers and insecurities, and seeking professional help when needed, couples can overcome obstacles and cultivate a more romantic and intimate sexual relationship.

Cheryl Bach

X.

Maintaining Romance in the Long Term

Maintaining romance in a long-term relationship requires effort and intentionality, especially as the dynamics of the relationship evolve over time. In this chapter, we'll explore strategies for keeping the romance alive, reinventing your sexual connection, and cultivating gratitude and appreciation for your partner.

A. Strategies for Keeping the Romance Alive as the Relationship Evolves

Prioritize Quality Time: Make time for regular date nights and activities that you both enjoy. Spending quality time together helps to strengthen your bond and keep the romance alive.

Surprise Each Other: Keep things exciting by surprising your partner with thoughtful gestures, gifts, or spontaneous acts of affection. Surprise dates, love notes, or small gestures of kindness can go a long way in keeping the spark alive.

Communicate Openly: Keep the lines of communication open by regularly checking in with each other and expressing your feelings and desires openly and honestly. Communication is key to maintaining emotional intimacy and connection.

Keep the Passion Alive: Don't let physical intimacy fall by the wayside. Make an effort to keep the passion alive by initiating sex, exploring new techniques and fantasies, and prioritizing pleasure and satisfaction for both partners.

B. Reinventing Your Sexual Connection over Time

Embrace Change: Recognize that sexual desire and preferences may change over time, and be open to exploring new ways of connecting sexually with your partner. Embrace change as an opportunity for growth and discovery in your relationship.

Try New Things: Keep your sexual relationship exciting and fulfilling by trying new activities, positions, and techniques together. Be open to exploring each other's fantasies and desires and finding creative ways to incorporate them into your sex life.

Keep Communicating: As your sexual relationship evolves, continue to communicate openly and honestly with your partner about your needs, desires, and boundaries. Regularly check in with each other to ensure that you're both feeling fulfilled and satisfied.

Cheryl Bach

Seek Inspiration: Draw inspiration from books, articles, workshops, or online resources that focus on sexual intimacy and pleasure. Educating yourselves and seeking out new ideas can help to keep your sexual connection fresh and exciting over time.

C. Cultivating Gratitude and Appreciation for Your Partner

Express Appreciation: Take time to express gratitude and appreciation for your partner regularly. Acknowledge their efforts, strengths, and qualities that you admire, and let them know how much they mean to you.

Practice Acts of Kindness: Show your partner that you care by performing small acts of kindness and thoughtfulness. Whether it's making them breakfast in bed, writing them a love letter, or simply giving them a heartfelt compliment, these gestures can strengthen your connection and deepen your bond.

Focus on the Positive: Make a conscious effort to focus on the positive aspects of your relationship and your partner. Cultivate an attitude of gratitude and look for opportunities to celebrate and cherish the love you share.

Celebrate Milestones: Take time to celebrate important milestones and anniversaries in your relationship. Whether it's your first date, your wedding anniversary, or the anniversary of a significant moment in your relationship, use these occasions as opportunities to reflect on your journey together and reaffirm your commitment to each other.

By implementing strategies for keeping the romance alive, reinventing your sexual connection, and cultivating gratitude and appreciation for your partner, you can maintain a romantic and intimate relationship that continues to thrive and grow over time.

Cheryl Bach

XI.
Conclusion

In this final chapter, we'll recap the key points discussed in this book, encourage couples to prioritize romance and intimacy in their sexual relationship, and offer some final words of advice for embarking on a journey towards more fulfilling and romantic sex.

A. Recap of Key Points Discussed in the Book

Throughout this book, we've explored various strategies and tips for making sex more romantic and intimate for couples.

Here's a recap of the key points discussed:

- Understanding the importance of romance and intimacy in sexual relationships.

- Building emotional connection through communication, quality time, and trust.

Cheryl Bach

- Creating a romantic atmosphere through ambiance and sensory experiences.

- Enhancing physical intimacy through non-sexual touch, cuddling, and massage.

- Spicing up foreplay with different activities and techniques.

- Trying new things together to keep the spark alive and deepen emotional connection.

- Overcoming common challenges such as stress, communication barriers, and insecurities.

- Maintaining romance in the long term by prioritizing quality time, reinventing sexual connection, and cultivating gratitude and appreciation for your partner.

B. Encouragement for Couples to Prioritize Romance and Intimacy

As you embark on this journey towards more fulfilling and romantic sex, we encourage you to prioritize romance and intimacy in your sexual relationship. Remember that maintaining a strong and satisfying connection with your partner requires effort, intentionality, and a willingness to explore and grow together.

Make time for each other, communicate openly and honestly, and be willing to try new things and experiment with different techniques and activities. Keep the passion alive by prioritizing physical intimacy and prioritizing pleasure and satisfaction for both partners.

By prioritizing romance and intimacy in your sexual relationship, you can deepen your emotional connection, strengthen your bond as a couple, and create a more fulfilling and satisfying sex life.

C. Final Words of Advice for Embarking on a Journey towards More Fulfilling and Romantic Sex

As you continue on your journey towards more fulfilling and romantic sex, remember to be patient with yourselves and with each other. Rome wasn't built in a day, and neither is a deeply satisfying sexual relationship. Take the time to explore, experiment, and grow together, and don't be afraid to seek help or guidance if you encounter challenges along the way.

Above all, remember that the most important ingredient in a fulfilling and romantic sex life is love and mutual respect. Treat each other with kindness, compassion, and understanding, and approach your sexual relationship with curiosity, enthusiasm, and a sense of adventure.

We hope that this book has provided you with valuable insights, inspiration, and practical tips for enhancing romance and intimacy in your sexual relationship. May your journey towards more fulfilling and romantic sex be filled with love, passion, and joy.

Cheryl Bach